1

DISCLAIMER

This book's content is only intended for general informative purposes. At the time of writing, the author has taken every precaution to guarantee that the material is correct and current. Nevertheless, the author disclaims all explicit and implicit representations and guarantees about the availability, appropriateness, correctness, completeness, and usefulness of the material on these pages.

Since the author is not a licensed medical practitioner, the material in this book shouldn't be interpreted as medical advice. Before making any modifications to their diet, exercise regimen, or medical treatment, readers are urged to speak with a licensed healthcare provider.

Moreover, the author has no connection to any of the businesses, organizations, or people that are discussed in this book. Any mentions of goods, services, businesses, or people are purely informative and do not indicate endorsement or suggestion.

This book's content is entirely dependent on the author's expertise, study, and comprehension of the topic. Despite having taken reasonable care to offer correct information, the author disclaims all liability for any mistakes or omissions in the material as well as for any losses, harm, or damages resulting from using the information.

It is recommended that readers use their own judgment and discretion when applying the knowledge in this book to their own situations. The use or implementation of any material in this book may result in unfavorable repercussions, directly or indirectly, for which the author assumes no liability.

By reading this book, you agree to release and hold the author harmless from any claims, losses, liabilities, costs, or expenditures resulting from or related to the use of the information you get from it.

Table of Contents

ABOUT THE BOOK

Not only a book, "Small Intestinal Bacterial Overgrowth" is an all-inclusive manual that provides the answers to comprehending, treating, and thriving with SIBO. With a thorough examination of every aspect of this illness, from its causes to doable lifestyle modifications, this book becomes a vital resource for anybody living with SIBO or helping someone who does.

The basics of SIBO are covered in Chapter 1, along with information on its causes, nature, and warning signs. This fundamental understanding creates the framework for wise choices and successful management techniques.

The complex world of the gut microbiome is introduced in Chapter 2, with special emphasis on its vital role in general health and how SIBO upsets this delicate equilibrium. Equipped with this knowledge, readers see why controlling SIBO necessitates restoring gut health.

The next chapters provide a road map for long-term maintenance, diagnosis, and treatment. Readers have insight into negotiating the challenges of treating SIBO from Chapter 3's interpretation of diagnostic tests to Chapter 4's examination of various treatment choices. The comprehensive discussion of dietary adjustments, antibiotic medication, herbal supplements, and lifestyle modifications provides readers with a variety of options catered to their specific requirements.

To empower readers to make educated dietary decisions, Chapter 6 offers helpful advice on meal planning, while Chapter 7 examines the function of probiotics and prebiotics in repairing gut health.

Chapters 8 and 9 address the psychological as well as the physical effects of SIBO and provide techniques for symptom management, recurrence prevention, and general well-being maintenance. Ultimately, Chapter 10 provides priceless advice on how to identify support systems and navigate social settings to build empowerment and resilience in the face of SIBO.

"Small Intestinal Bacterial Overgrowth" is a lifeline for anybody trying to reclaim control over their health and quality of life in the face of this difficult illness, rather than just a book. It is an invaluable companion on the path to health because of its thorough coverage, sensible guidance, and kind demeanor.

CHAPTER 1

Understanding Small Intestinal Bacterial Overgrowth (Sibo)

What Is Sibo?

An abnormal rise in the number of bacteria in the small intestine is known as small intestinal bacterial overgrowth or SIBO. The majority of the body's gut bacteria dwell in the large intestine, which typically has a higher concentration of bacteria than the small intestine. But with SIBO, bacteria overgrow or migrate from the large intestine into the small intestine, causing a host of digestive disorders as well as other health concerns.

Causes Of Sibo

Effective management and treatment of SIBO depend on an understanding of its etiology. SIBO may arise as a result of many factors:

1. **Reduced Gut motility:** Food and waste are moved through the digestive system by the muscles of the tract. Bacterial accumulation in the small intestine may result from malfunctioning of these muscles.

2. **Structural Abnormalities:** Disorders such as intestinal strictures or diverticula, which are tiny pouches that may develop in the walls of the intestines, can provide pockets in which bacteria can grow and multiply.

3. **Low Stomach Acid:** The acid in our stomachs is essential for eliminating dangerous microorganisms from the food we consume. Bacteria that enter the small intestine may thrive and multiply if there is little stomach acid.

4. **Immune System Weakness:** Bacterial overgrowth in the small intestine may be difficult to successfully manage if the immune system is compromised.

5. Certain Medical Conditions: SIBO risk may be elevated by conditions including diabetes, celiac disease, and Crohn's disease.

6. Medication: Certain drugs, especially those that impact stomach acid production or intestinal motility, might make people more susceptible to SIBO.

Symptoms To Look Out For

Early identification and treatment of SIBO depend on the ability to identify its symptoms. While each person's symptoms may differ, frequent indicators of SIBO include:

1. Bloating, gas, cramps, and abdominal pain are examples of abdominal discomfort. After eating, these feelings often become worse, particularly with meals heavy in carbs.

2. Constipation or diarrhea: SIBO may interfere with regular bowel movements, resulting in either difficulty passing stools or a lot of loose stools.

3. Nutritional deficits: SIBO-related malabsorption of nutrients may result in vitamin and mineral deficits, including iron and B12.

4. Weariness: One typical SIBO symptom is chronic weariness, which is probably brought on by the body's immune system reacting to bacterial overgrowth and nutritional loss.

5. Weight Loss: Unintentional weight loss may happen as a result of altered appetite and nutritional malabsorption.

6. Additional Symptoms: These might include headaches, skin rashes, joint discomfort, and acid reflux, among others.

CHAPTER 2

The Gut Microbiome

Introduction To The Gut Microbiome

The intestines are the primary home of a large ecosystem of bacteria known as the gut microbiome. The gut microbiota is the aggregate term for billions of bacteria, viruses, fungi, and other microorganisms that make up this ecosystem. These microorganisms are essential to our digestion, immunity, metabolism, and even mental well-being, among other elements of our health.

There is a fine balance between helpful and detrimental microbes in the gut microbiome. A disturbance in this equilibrium may result in several health problems, such as SIBO (small intestine bacterial overgrowth).

For this reason, it is crucial to maintain a varied and healthy gut microbiota for general health and well-being.

Importance Of A Healthy Gut

For appropriate digestion and food absorption, a healthy gut is essential. Complex carbs, fiber, and other nutrients that the body is unable to absorb on its own are broken down by the gut microbiota. These microorganisms also create vital vitamins, such as vitamin K and several B vitamins, which are important for several body processes.

Furthermore, the immune system is greatly assisted by the gut flora. The gut-associated lymphoid tissue (GALT), where they interact with the gut microbiota, is home to around 70% of the body's immune cells. An immune system that is in balance is better able to control inflammation and infections.

Furthermore, new studies indicate that the gut-brain axis may be a mechanism by which the gut microbiota influences mental health and cognitive performance. Changes in the gut microbiota may affect brain function and vice versa due to the bidirectional signaling that occurs within the communication network between the gut and the brain. This link emphasizes how crucial it is to keep your gut healthy to have the best possible mental health.

How Sibo Impacts The Gut Microbiome

An unnatural rise in the number of bacteria in the small intestine is known as small intestinal bacterial overgrowth or SIBO. In comparison to the large intestine, the small intestine typically has a lower bacterial population. But with SIBO, colon bacteria either move or multiply excessively inside the small intestine, resulting in symptoms related to the digestive system as well as other health issues.

SIBO induces an overgrowth of bacteria in the small intestine, upsetting the delicate equilibrium of the gut microbiome. This overgrowth may result in bloating and excessive gas production, as well as poor digestion and nutritional absorption. Furthermore, bacteria in the small intestine may harm the intestinal lining, causing inflammation and aggravating symptoms related to digestion.

Moreover, SIBO may affect immunological response, metabolism, and even mental health in addition to gastrointestinal health. An overabundance of bacteria in the small intestine may lead to inflammation and immunological reactions, which can aggravate a variety of bodily conditions. Furthermore, methane and hydrogen sulfide, two bacterial byproducts generated in SIBO, may be neurotoxic and impair cognitive function.

SIBO disturbs the gut flora and may have a significant impact on immunological response, digestive health, and general well-being. The goal of managing SIBO is to improve health outcomes and reduce symptoms by re-establishing the balance of the gut microbiome using targeted therapies such as probiotics, antibiotics, and dietary changes.

CHAPTER 3

Diagnosis Of Sibo

Common Diagnostic Tests

Several tests are used to diagnose small intestinal bacterial overgrowth (SIBO), which is a condition caused by an overabundance of bacteria in the small intestine. Among the most popular tests are:

1. **Breath Tests:** A common non-invasive method for diagnosing SIBO is the breath test. If the bacteria are present in the small intestine, the patient takes a substrate such as glucose or lactulose, which is fermented by them. Gases like hydrogen and methane are produced by bacteria during the fermentation of these substrates, and the breath is used to monitor these gases. Bacterial overgrowth is indicated by elevated amounts of these gasses.

2. Aspirate Culture: During this process, a medical professional puts a tube down the nose and into the small intestine to take a fluid sample. After that, the fluid is cultivated to determine and measure the types of bacteria present. Aspirate cultures provide immediate proof of bacterial proliferation, albeit being more intrusive.

3. Small Bowel Aspirate: This test, which is comparable to aspirate culture, involves putting a tube into the small intestine to collect a sample for examination. It's often carried out in conjunction with an endoscopy.

4. Blood Tests: To look for indicators of malabsorption, inflammatory conditions, or nutritional deficits that may be connected to SIBO, blood tests may be performed. Increased concentrations of certain indicators, such as folate, vitamin B12, or inflammatory markers, might point to SIBO as a potential culprit.

5. **Stool testing:** Although less often used to diagnose SIBO, stool testing may provide details about the general balance of gut bacteria and identify any abnormalities that could be linked to the illness.

Interpreting Test Results

Healthcare personnel need to have specialized knowledge to interpret the findings of SIBO diagnostic tests. SIBO is indicated by elevated hydrogen and/or methane levels in breath tests or by the presence of certain bacterial species in aspirate cultures. To establish the diagnosis, it's crucial to take into account other variables including symptoms, medical history, and test findings.

Usually, breath tests evaluate the gas levels after swallowing a substrate at many different times. An increase in gas during a certain period points to small intestinal bacterial overgrowth.

False positives or negatives, however, may happen for several reasons, including medicine, food, or underlying medical disorders that impact gut motility.

High concentrations of bacteria, especially coliform bacteria like Escherichia coli, Streptococcus species, and Staphylococcus aureus, are indicative of SIBO in aspirate cultures. However, to differentiate between normal and pathogenic bacteria concentrations, microbiological competence is required for the interpretation of culture findings.

Blood testing may identify anomalies such as SIBO-associated inflammation or nutritional deficits. The diagnosis may be supported by elevated levels of inflammatory markers such as C-reactive protein (CRP) vitamin B12, folate, or both.

Stool testing may provide further information about the makeup of the gut microbiota and any dysbiosis that could be a factor in SIBO. Disproportions between good and bad bacteria, together with indicators of infection or inflammation, might point to SIBO as a potential source of gastrointestinal problems.

Consulting With Healthcare Professionals

It is essential to speak with medical experts to correctly diagnose and treat SIBO. Individualized treatment regimens may be created for patients by gastroenterologists, internists, or functional medicine professionals who specialize in gastrointestinal problems.

Patients should give a thorough medical history, including symptoms, food, medicines, and any prior diagnostic testing or therapies, before seeking medical guidance for suspected SIBO. Based on the patient's symptoms and medical history, medical practitioners may suggest certain tests to confirm or rule out SIBO.

Healthcare providers talk with patients about test findings, their consequences, and possible treatment choices during consultations. In addition, they could answer any worries or inquiries patients might have about SIBO, its causes, and its treatment options.

When SIBO is verified, medical experts collaborate closely with patients to create customized treatment regimens that suit their requirements and preferences. To address underlying reasons and relieve symptoms, treatment options may include probiotics, antibiotic medication, dietary alterations, and lifestyle adjustments.

Scheduling regular follow-up sessions enables medical staff to keep an eye on patients' progress, make any adjustments to treatment plans, and handle any emerging symptoms or concerns. Through successful management of SIBO and enhanced quality of life, patients may work with skilled and experienced healthcare experts.

CHAPTER 4

Treatment Options

Dietary Changes For Managing Sibo

Overview of Dietary Adjustments: The first line of treatment for Small Intestinal Bacterial Overgrowth (SIBO) is often dietary modification. The aim is to provide an environment in the intestines that inhibits the development of germs and lessens symptoms like gas, bloating, and discomfort in the abdomen.

Low FODMAP Diet: The Low FODMAP (Fermentable Oligosaccharides, Disaccharides, Monosaccharides, and Polyols) diet is one of the dietary strategies for SIBO that is most often advised. Foods that are heavy in certain kinds of carbs, which may ferment in the stomach and worsen symptoms, are avoided on this diet.

Goods rich in fructooligosaccharides (FODMAPs) include certain fruits, vegetables, grains, and legumes.

Specific Carbohydrate Diet (SCD): The Specific Carbohydrate Diet (SCD) is an additional dietary strategy that may help control SIBO. Complex carbs like those found in grains, certain sweets, and the majority of dairy products are restricted in this diet. Reducing the amount of carbohydrates that are available to feed bacteria in the small intestine is the aim.

Elemental Diet: For the management of SIBO, medical professionals may sometimes suggest an elemental diet. This is ingesting liquid nutrients that have already been partially digested. These nutrients are taken higher up in the digestive system, avoiding the small intestine, which is the site of bacterial overgrowth.

Although beneficial, following an elemental diet may be difficult and may need medical monitoring.

Prebiotics and Probiotics: Probiotics are good bacteria that may aid in reestablishing the gut microbiota's equilibrium. On the other hand, adding more bacteria can make SIBO symptoms worse. Additionally, because prebiotics may fuel the overgrowth of bacteria in the small intestine, they should be avoided. Prebiotics are chemicals that encourage the development of good bacteria.

Customized Approach: It's crucial to remember that dietary guidelines for treating SIBO might change based on a person's symptoms, underlying medical issues, and reaction to certain foods. Personalized dietary advice and optimal symptom management may be achieved by collaborating with a gastrointestinal health specialist or dietitian.

Antibiotic Therapy

Overview of Antibiotic treatment: By focusing on and lowering the number of bacteria in the small intestine, antibiotic treatment is often used to treat Small Intestinal Bacterial Overgrowth (SIBO). To reduce the danger of antibiotic resistance and other negative consequences, antibiotic treatment should be used carefully and under a doctor's supervision.

Rifaximin is a non-absorbable antibiotic that is often used to treat small intestine bleeding (SIBO). To minimize systemic adverse effects, it exclusively targets bacteria in the stomach without entering the circulation. It has been shown that rifaximin works well to lessen SIBO symptoms such as gas, bloating, and stomach discomfort.

Other Antibiotics: Metronidazole, neomycin, and ciprofloxacin are a few other antibiotics that may be taken alone or in combination to treat SIBO, in addition to rifaximin. The kind of bacteria present, the intensity of the symptoms, and the patient's reaction to therapy all play a role in the antibiotic selection process.

Treatment Duration: Depending on the underlying reason for bacterial overgrowth and the patient's reaction to treatment, the length of antibiotic therapy for SIBO may vary. A brief course of antibiotics may be enough to alleviate symptoms in certain situations, while intermittent or long-term therapy may be required in others to avoid recurrence.

Combination Therapy: To relieve symptoms and stop recurrence in situations with resistant or recurrent SIBO, combination therapy combining numerous antibiotics or antibiotics with additional therapeutic modalities such as dietary modifications or prokinetic drugs may be required.

Monitoring and Follow-up: To evaluate treatment response, keep an eye out for side effects, and make necessary medication adjustments, regular monitoring and follow-up with a healthcare professional are crucial throughout antibiotic therapy for SIBO. To reduce the chance of recurrence, it's crucial to take antibiotics as directed for the whole recommended course, even if symptoms subside before it's over.

Herbal Supplements And Alternative Therapies

Overview of Herbal Supplements and Alternative Therapies: Some people with Small Intestinal Bacterial Overgrowth (SIBO) may consider herbal supplements and alternative therapies as supplemental or adjunctive methods to manage their symptoms, in addition to traditional treatments like diet modifications and antibiotic therapy.

Herbal Antibiotics: A few herbal supplements include antibacterial qualities that might aid in lowering the amount of bacteria that overgrows in the small intestine. Garlic extract, grapefruit seed extract, oregano oil, and berberine are a few examples. Depending on the severity of the symptoms and personal preferences, these herbal medicines may be administered either on their own or in conjunction with traditional antibiotics.

Prokinetic Agents: Prokinetic agents are drugs or dietary supplements that enhance the motility of the gastrointestinal tract and stop food and germs from becoming stuck in the small intestine. plant prokinetics may help with digestion and lessen SIBO symptoms. Examples of these are ginger, peppermint oil, and Iberogast, which is a blend of many plant extracts.

Digestive Enzymes: Food molecules may be broken down into smaller, easier-to-digest parts with the aid of digestive enzymes. Digestive enzyme supplements may help people with SIBO digest food better and absorb nutrients more easily, which can lessen symptoms like bloating and pain in the abdomen.

Nutrients for Gut Healing: Some nutrients are believed to help mend the intestinal lining, which may be damaged in SIBO patients, and promote gut health. These consist of aloe vera, zinc carnosine, glutamine, and deglycyrrhizinated licorice (DGL). Nevertheless, there is little data to support the use of these supplements in the treatment of SIBO, therefore care should be taken while using them.

Consultation with Healthcare Provider: It's crucial to get advice from a healthcare professional, especially one who specializes in gastrointestinal health, before beginning any herbal supplements or other treatments for SIBO. Before beginning therapy, it's important to go over the possible dangers and advantages of using any herbal supplements since some may combine with drugs or worsen underlying health concerns. Furthermore, the quality and purity of herbal supplements might differ between goods since they are not subject to the same regulations as pharmaceutical pharmaceuticals.

CHAPTER 5

Lifestyle Modifications

Stress Management Techniques

Stress has a major negative effect on gut health and exacerbates diseases such as SIBO (small intestine bacterial overgrowth). Using practical stress-reduction strategies is essential for controlling SIBO symptoms and enhancing general well-being.

Mindfulness meditation is one useful method. This is directing your attention to the here and now, without passing judgment. People may manage their stress levels and better handle SIBO symptoms by practicing mindfulness. Frequent meditation, even for a little while each day, may have a big impact.

Exercises including deep breathing are another beneficial tactic. The body's relaxation response, which is triggered by deep breathing, offsets the physiological consequences of stress. People with SIBO may reduce their pain by using deep breathing methods like square breathing or diaphragmatic breathing to relax their nervous system.

Meditation and tai chi are examples of relaxation-promoting exercises that may help with stress management and intestinal health. These techniques encourage both mental and physical relaxation by combining breath awareness with gentle movement. Regular yoga or tai chi practice may help you feel less stressed and improve your quality of life in general.

In addition, using healthy coping strategies like journaling, going outside, or interacting with loved ones might provide resilience and emotional support while dealing with SIBO-related difficulties. People may improve their well-being and better manage their conditions by learning and using appropriate stress management practices.

Importance Of Regular Exercise

Maintaining general gut health and controlling Small Intestinal Bacterial Overgrowth (SIBO) depend heavily on regular exercise. Exercise has been shown to boost immunity, decrease inflammation, and increase intestinal motility—all of which are advantageous for those who have SIBO.

Walking, running, or cycling are examples of aerobic activity that may help promote bowel movements and keep the small intestine from becoming stagnant, which lowers the risk of bacterial overgrowth. Strength training activities that increase muscle mass and metabolic function, such as weightlifting or resistance training, may also benefit intestinal health.

Exercise has a direct impact on gut health, but it also helps reduce stress, which is a significant cause of SIBO symptoms. Exercising causes the body to produce endorphins, which are feel-good and stress-relieving neurotransmitters. Regular exercise may help you become more resilient to stress and effectively manage the symptoms associated with SIBO.

Finding hobbies you like and can stick with over time is key. The important thing is to be active and prioritize fitness in your life, whether that means dancing, swimming, or participating in sports. Most days of the week, try to get in at least 30 minutes of moderate-intensity activity. As your fitness level increases, progressively up the time and intensity.

Always pay attention to your body and adjust your workout regimen to suit any limits or symptoms associated with SIBO. A certified fitness teacher or a member of the medical community may provide you with advice on creating a safe and efficient exercise program that fits your requirements and objectives.

Sleep Hygiene For Gut Health

Getting enough sleep is crucial for gut health and general well-being, particularly for those who have SIBO (small intestine bacterial overgrowth). It's critical to emphasize sleep hygiene habits since getting too little sleep may interfere with immune system function, upset the body's circadian cycles, and worsen digestive problems.

Promoting good sleep patterns requires establishing a regular sleep routine. To keep your body's internal clock in check, try to go to bed and get up at the same time every day—even on the weekends. Establishing a calming nighttime routine, like reading a book, having a warm bath, or doing relaxation exercises, might help your body know when it's time to wind down and get ready for sleep.

Making your space conducive to rest might also improve the quality of your slumber. Maintain a cool, quiet, and dark bedroom. To enhance sleep comfort, choose a good mattress and pillows. Reduce the amount of time spent in front of a screen before going to bed. The blue light that these gadgets generate may disrupt the body's natural synthesis of melatonin, a hormone that controls sleep-wake cycles. Examples of such devices are laptops, tablets, and smartphones.

Reducing stimulating activities before bed, such as large meals, coffee, and strenuous exercise, may also aid in improving sleep quality.

Alternatively, go for light food and relaxing herbal teas. To determine the underlying causes of your insomnia or other sleep disorders and create a customized treatment plan, think about speaking with a healthcare provider.

Making sleep a priority in your life and emphasizing sleep hygiene routines can help you manage SIBO-related symptoms, maintain gut health, and enhance your general well-being.

CHAPTER 6

Meal Planning For Sibo

Sibo-Friendly Foods

When it comes to treating Small Intestinal Bacterial Overgrowth (SIBO), dietary selection is crucial. Reducing the amount of fermentable carbohydrates consumed is the aim since they might worsen symptoms by providing food for the proliferating bacteria in the small intestine. Foods low in fermentable carbs tend to be more well-tolerated and trigger flare-ups less often.

Lean meats, poultry, fish, and eggs are examples of foods that are SIBO-friendly. In addition to being low in fermentable carbs, these meals include vital nutrients like protein and amino acids, which are critical for maintaining muscle mass and general health.

Furthermore, proteins tend to be more filling, which might aid in regulating appetite and avoiding overindulging.

Spinach, kale, bell peppers, and other non-starchy vegetables make up another category of SIBO-friendly meals. These veggies are low in fermentable carbs and high in vitamins, minerals, and antioxidants, which makes them good options for those with SIBO. It's crucial to pay attention to portion proportions, too, since eating a lot of veggies might sometimes exacerbate symptoms.

Many people with SIBO may also handle healthy fats, such as those in nuts, seeds, avocados, and olive oil. When included in meals, these fats provide a concentrated source of energy and may support the sensation of fullness. They may also improve the absorption of fat-soluble vitamins, which is advantageous for those whose SIBO has impeded their ability to absorb nutrients.

Lastly, some people with SIBO may eat low-sugar foods in moderation, such as citrus fruits and berries. These fruits provide a range of vitamins and minerals along with their natural sweetness, all without dramatically raising the consumption of fermentable carbs. Nonetheless, because some individuals may be more sensitive to certain fruit varieties than others, it's critical to keep an eye on symptoms and modify fruit diet appropriately.

In conclusion, meals high in healthy fats, low in sugar fruits, and non-starchy veggies are all SIBO-friendly. SIBO sufferers may improve their general health and well-being and more effectively control their symptoms by concentrating on these food categories and reducing their consumption of fermentable carbs.

Meal Preparation Tips

Preparing meals helps people manage their SIBO because it gives them more control over the components and serving sizes of their meals, which lowers the chance of flare-ups. Here are some useful hints for cooking meals that are SIBO-friendly:

1. Make a plan: Set aside some time each week to organize your snacks and meals. When hunger hits, this may help you make healthy decisions rather than grabbing for quick, less nourishing alternatives. To make the process go more smoothly, think about creating a weekly grocery list and meal plan.

2. Emphasis on entire Foods: Whenever feasible, choose entire, minimally processed foods. When compared to processed foods, they generally have more nutrients and less fermentable carbs.

Choose nutritious grains like brown rice and quinoa, lean meats, and healthy fats.

3. Cook from Scratch: When you make your food, you can maintain control over the ingredients and steer clear of sneaky sources of fermentable carbs like added sugars and preservatives. To add variation to your meals, try experimenting with various cooking techniques including roasting, grilling, steaming, and sautéing.

4. Use SIBO-Friendly Substitutes: To make your favorite meals more SIBO-friendly, be inventive when it comes to ingredient replacements. For instance, use zucchini noodles instead of wheat spaghetti, change out cow's milk with lactose-free options like almond or coconut milk, and substitute cauliflower rice for regular rice.

5. Practice Portion Control: Be mindful of the amounts you consume to prevent overindulging, which may further tax your digestive system. To properly measure out your meals, particularly when preparing grains, legumes, and high-starch veggies, use measuring cups, spoons, or a food scale.

6. Think About Meal Timing: For some people with SIBO, distributing meals and snacks evenly throughout the day aids with symptom management. For stable blood sugar levels and to avoid too much fermentation in the small intestine, try to eat every three to four hours.

7. Be Aware of meal pairings: Some meal pairings might impact digestion and make SIBO symptoms worse in sufferers. For instance, eating high-fat and high-carbohydrate diets together may cause bacterial overgrowth and delay stomach emptying. Try a variety of meal combinations to see what suits you the best.

Sample Meal Plans

These meal prep suggestions will help you make scrumptious, wholesome meals that can improve your health and help you properly manage SIBO symptoms.

Example Menus

Making healthy, filling meals doesn't have to be difficult while dealing with SIBO. Here are some examples of meal plans to get you going:

First Sample Meal Plan:

• Eggs scrambled with spinach and cherry tomatoes for breakfast

• Snack: cucumber slices and Greek yogurt

• Lunch would be grilled chicken salad dressed with a balsamic vinaigrette, mixed greens, and avocado.

• Snack: Rice cakes with almond butter

• Supper is baked salmon over quinoa and roasted asparagus.

Second Sample Meal Plan:

• Smoothie made with protein powder, spinach, berries, and almond milk for breakfast.

• Snack: Hummus-topped carrot sticks

• Turkey lettuce wraps with salsa, bell peppers, and avocado for lunch

• Snack: Almonds and seeds combined

• Dinner is cauliflower rice, broccoli, and bell peppers stir-fried with tofu.

You are welcome to alter these meal plans to suit your dietary needs, food intolerances, and personal tastes.

CHAPTER 7

Probiotics And Prebiotics

Understanding Probiotics And Prebiotics

Probiotics and prebiotics provide a safe and efficient means of restoring the proper balance of gut flora and are crucial weapons in the fight against Small Intestinal Bacterial Overgrowth (SIBO). Let's explore the meaning of these phrases and how they affect the health of your digestive system.

Prebiotics

Probiotics are living bacteria that provide the host health advantages when taken in sufficient doses. These good bacteria support the restoration of your gut microbiome's delicate equilibrium, which is often upset by illnesses like SIBO. Probiotics help reduce SIBO symptoms like bloating, gas, and pain in the abdomen by crowding out bad bacteria in your system and increasing the number of "good" bacteria.

It's important to take the potency and strain specificity into account when choosing probiotic pills. Selecting a probiotic supplement that includes strains of bacteria that are beneficial against SIBO is crucial since different probiotic strains have different impacts on gut health. Seek for items that have a high colony-forming unit (CFU) count to make sure you're receiving enough good bacteria.

Probiotics

Prebiotics are indigestible fibers that act as food for probiotics in your stomach, promoting their growth and multiplication. Prebiotics provide your body with the nutrition that probiotics supply so that the good bacteria may grow and thrive. You may provide the ideal conditions for probiotics to colonize and start working their magic by adding foods high in prebiotics to your diet or taking prebiotic supplements.

Whole grains, some fruits, and vegetables are common sources of prebiotics. These meals include fibers such as resistant starches, oligosaccharides, and inulin that pass through the digestive system undigested and encourage the colon's good bacteria to proliferate. You may encourage the growth of probiotics and improve the health of your gut by including a range of foods high in prebiotics in your diet.

How They Benefit Gut Health

There are several advantages to probiotics and prebiotics for gut health, especially when SIBO is present. Together, they support a healthy digestive tract and reduce SIBO symptoms in the following ways:

Because SIBO upsets the delicate equilibrium of bacteria in the small intestine, good bacteria are depleted and bad bacteria proliferate. By bringing good bacteria into the stomach, driving away harmful bacteria, and increasing microbial diversity, probiotics aid in the restoration of this equilibrium. Prebiotics provide probiotics with the nutrition they need to grow, which improves colonization and efficacy.

Diminishing Manifestations

Bloating, gas, diarrhea, and stomach discomfort are just a few of the symptoms of SIBO that may seriously lower your quality of life. Probiotics have been shown to improve digestion, lower inflammation, and restore gut motility to ease these symptoms. By encouraging the development of good bacteria that generate short-chain fatty acids, which have anti-inflammatory and protective properties for the gut lining, prebiotics enhance the benefits of probiotics.

Boosting Immune Response

A strong immune system depends on a healthy gut microbiota since it is critical for controlling immunological responses and protecting the body from infections. By increasing the activity of immune cells and encouraging the generation of anti-inflammatory cytokines, probiotics aid in immune system modulation. By encouraging the development of good bacteria that interact with the immune system and support a balanced immunological response, prebiotics boosts the health of the immune system.

Choosing The Right Supplements

Probiotics and prebiotics should be chosen carefully for controlling SIBO. Make sure the supplements are of a good caliber, supported by research, and designed to work. These pointers will help you choose the appropriate supplements:

Search for Particular Strains

Certain probiotic strains may work better than others to treat SIBO since they are not all made equal. Seek supplements that include strains that have been shown to reduce SIBO symptoms and decrease the development of harmful bacteria, such as Lactobacillus acidophilus, Bifidobacterium bifidum, and Saccharomyces boulardii.

Think about CFU Count

Probiotic supplements are rated according to their potency using colony-forming units (CFUs), which represent the quantity of live bacteria in a given dosage. To be sure you're receiving a proper dosage of helpful bacteria, look for supplements with a high CFU count. Higher CFU counts are often connected with higher efficiency.

Seek supplements that have undergone independent testing to ensure their safety, efficacy, and purity. Select goods from reliable manufacturers that follow Good Manufacturing Practices (GMP) and have a history of creating high-quality dietary supplements. Third-party certifications, like USP Verified or NSF International, may provide an extra layer of quality and effectiveness assurance.

In summary, probiotics and prebiotics are essential for controlling SIBO and fostering gut health in general. For the best possible digestive health, you may relieve symptoms, boost your immune system, and restore microbial balance by including these nutrients in your daily routine and selecting high-quality goods.

CHAPTER 8

Managing Symptoms

Dealing With Digestive Discomfort

One of the most difficult aspects of having Small Intestinal Bacterial Overgrowth (SIBO) is dealing with digestive pain. It is essential to comprehend efficient symptom management if one hopes to enhance overall quality of life. Finding certain triggers that aggravate symptoms is one of the first stages in managing stomach pain. This may include certain meals, tension, or drugs.

Consuming food tailored to the needs of SIBOs is one way to alleviate intestinal distress. For the most part, this is cutting down on or giving up items that are known to make symptoms worse, such as high-food meals, dairy, gluten, and refined carbohydrates.

Alternatively, emphasizing meals that are readily digested, such as vegetables, low-sugar fruits, and lean meats, might help ease the pain.

Certain lifestyle adjustments may help manage stomach pain in addition to food changes. Deep breathing exercises, yoga, and other stress-reduction methods might help lower general stress levels, which may lessen SIBO symptoms. Frequent exercise may help lessen pain and support a healthy digestive system.

It could be required to use over-the-counter or prescription medicine for those who are suffering severe intestinal pain. Digestion enzymes may assist break down food and lessen bloating and gas, while probiotics can help reestablish a healthy balance of gut flora.

To successfully manage the digestive pain associated with SIBO, it is ultimately important to find the proper mix of dietary adjustments, lifestyle modifications, and medicines. Developing a personalized treatment plan that targets individual requirements and symptoms may be facilitated by close collaboration with a licensed dietician or healthcare professional.

Strategies For Bloating Relief

Bloating is a typical SIBO symptom that may be difficult and painful to manage. Thankfully, several methods might help relieve bloating and lessen its intensity.

Eating smaller, more frequent meals throughout the day is one efficient way to reduce bloating. This may lessen the chance of bloating after meals and keep the digestive tract from being overworked. Eating slowly and properly chewing food may also improve digestion and lessen the quantity of air that is ingested, both of which can cause bloating.

A few dietary adjustments may also help reduce SIBO-related bloating. Chewing gum, carbonated drinks, and other items that cause gas may be avoided to help lessen excess gas in the digestive system. Including high-fiber meals like fruits, vegetables, and whole grains may also help to encourage regular bowel movements and lessen bloating.

Certain over-the-counter drugs, including simethicone or gas relief pills, may occasionally provide momentary relief from bloating. Before starting any new medicine, you should speak with your doctor, particularly if you have any underlying medical issues or are already on medication.

If bloating is severe or chronic, it could be important to look into other treatments like herbal supplements or prescription drugs. Herbal therapies like ginger or peppermint oil may also assist relieve bloating and enhance intestinal motility. Prokinetic drugs may also aid.

Addressing Nutrient Deficiencies

Since the overgrowth of bacteria in the small intestine may interfere with the body's capacity to absorb nutrients efficiently, nutritional shortages are a significant issue for those with SIBO. It is essential to address these inadequacies if general health and well-being are to be preserved.

Vitamin B12 is one of the most crucial nutrients to keep an eye on in people with SIBO. Overgrowth of bacteria in the small intestine may hinder vitamin B12 absorption, which over time might result in a shortage. An insufficient amount of vitamin B12 may cause weakness, exhaustion, and neurological issues. Correcting the deficit and averting long-term problems may need vitamin B12 injections or oral supplements.

Another major issue for people with SIBO is iron insufficiency because bacteria in the small intestine might prevent the body from absorbing iron from the diet. Iron deficiency symptoms might include weakness, exhaustion, and dyspnea. It could be essential to take iron supplements to raise iron levels and reduce symptoms.

Apart from iron and vitamin B12, SIBO may also impact the following nutrients: zinc, calcium, magnesium, and vitamin D. A customized supplementing plan may be created by identifying deficiencies and collaborating with a healthcare physician or registered dietitian to monitor nutrient levels via blood testing.

Lean meats, fruits, vegetables, and whole grains are examples of nutrient-dense foods that may be included in the diet to enhance general health and reduce the chance of nutritional shortages.

CHAPTER 9

Long-Term Maintenance

Preventing Sibo Recurrence

After SIBO has been effectively treated, maintaining long-term health depends on avoiding its return. Even if total avoidance isn't always achievable, using certain tactics may greatly lower the risk of SIBO recurring.

First and foremost, eating a balanced diet is important. Bacterial overgrowth may be prevented by avoiding foods that are known to aggravate SIBO, such as refined sugars and meals rich in FODMAPs. Rather, concentrate on eating a well-balanced diet full of fiber, healthy fats, lean proteins, and whole foods. Fiber helps maintain a healthy digestive system and may guard against bacterial imbalances in the small intestine.

It is particularly found in fruits, vegetables, and whole grains.

Supplements could help avoid a recurrence of SIBO. By re-establishing the proper balance of good bacteria in the gut, probiotics that include strains of Lactobacillus and Bifidobacterium may help reduce the number of harmful species that thrive there. Furthermore, several minerals and herbs, including digestive enzymes, oregano oil, and berberine, may promote intestinal health and prevent the formation of germs.

Another important strategy for avoiding SIBO recurrence is to maintain healthy intestinal motility. Frequent exercise, such as yoga or walking, may aid in promoting digestive contractions and preventing food from becoming stagnant in the small intestine. By lessening the interruptions to digestion caused by stress, stress-reduction methods like meditation or deep breathing exercises may help support healthy gut function.

Finally, treating any underlying issues that could be putting you at risk for SIBO is crucial. This might include ailments including diabetes, hypothyroidism, or anatomical digestive system anomalies. Reducing the risk of SIBO recurrence may be achieved by carefully collaborating with your healthcare practitioner to address these problems properly.

Follow-Up Care And Monitoring

Following SIBO therapy, ongoing monitoring and care are necessary to make sure the illness doesn't return and to manage any residual symptoms. Usually, your healthcare physician will set up follow-up sessions to evaluate your progress and modify your treatment plan as needed.

Your doctor may run diagnostic tests during these follow-up visits to assess the condition of your digestive system and look for any indications of bacterial overgrowth. This might include blood testing to check for nutritional deficiencies or inflammatory indicators, as well as breath tests to evaluate hydrogen and methane levels.

It's important to pay attention to your body and any symptoms that can point to a return of SIBO in addition to professional evaluations. These could include gas, bloating, constipation, diarrhea, or stomach discomfort. Maintaining a symptom diary might assist you in monitoring any changes over time and provide your doctor with useful information.

Your doctor may suggest periodic maintenance therapy to stop SIBO recurrence based on your unique risk factors and treatment response. To promote digestive health, this may include continuing to take certain vitamins or drugs, altering one's diet, or changing one's way of living.

Incorporating Healthy Habits For Lasting Results

Maintaining the long-term effects of SIBO therapy requires you to incorporate healthy practices into your everyday routine. This entails adopting a proactive self-care approach in addition to making dietary and lifestyle modifications.

Begin by gradually altering your diet, emphasizing whole, high-nutrient meals that promote intestinal health. Try a variety of meals to find any triggers that can make your symptoms worse, and make sure your intake of macro and micronutrients is balanced.

Maintaining digestive health overall and intestinal motility also requires regular physical exercise. On most days of the week, try to get in at least 30 minutes of moderate activity. Make sure the exercises you choose fit into your lifestyle and are enjoyable.

Stress management must be prioritized in addition to diet and exercise to avoid SIBO recurrence. Engage in relaxation practices like yoga, meditation, or deep breathing to lower stress levels and encourage balance and tranquility.

Lastly, maintain regular check-ups and communication with your healthcare professional to ensure that any issues are addressed and your progress is tracked. By adopting these health-promoting behaviors into your everyday routine, you may help guarantee long-lasting outcomes and lower your chance of experiencing another SIBO episode.

CHAPTER 10

Living Well With Sibo

Navigating Social Situations

Living with Small Intestinal Bacterial Overgrowth (SIBO) may bring particular difficulties in social settings, but you can confidently handle these circumstances if you have certain tactics and knowledge. For those with SIBO, juggling dietary restrictions with social engagements is one of the biggest challenges. It's important to let friends, family, and hosts know in advance about your dietary requirements so that there are alternatives that won't make your symptoms worse.

When eating out or attending events, it's beneficial to look up the menu ahead of time if at all feasible. Seek for recipes that are low in fermentable carbs (FODMAPs) and inquire about possible adjustments to meet your dietary requirements. Do not be afraid to ask the waitress or chef for clarification if you have questions about any particular ingredients. Recall that it's OK to put your health first and speak out for yourself.

Pacing oneself at social gatherings is crucial, in addition to taking care of nutritional issues. Overeating or ingesting trigger foods may cause SIBO symptoms to flare up, so pay attention to your body's needs and engage in mindful eating. If there aren't many appropriate meal alternatives, think about packing portable snacks or mini snacks. Being proactive and organizing ahead of time can allow you to attend social events without sacrificing your well-being.

Support Networks And Resources

Developing a robust support system is essential for treating SIBO and preserving general health. Friends, relatives, or online forums are all excellent resources for finding others who can relate to and understand your experience. Look for forums or support groups where you may talk to others who are facing comparable difficulties. It may help to reduce feelings of loneliness and give you the confidence to take charge of your health by exchanging experiences, advice, and support.

Professional resources may also help control SIBO, in addition to peer assistance. Think about collaborating with a medical professional who specializes in digestive issues, such as a functional medicine practitioner or gastroenterologist. They may assist in creating a customized treatment plan that is suited to your unique requirements and track your advancement over time. Furthermore, qualified dietitians with knowledge of digestive health may provide advice on dietary changes and nutritional tactics for efficient symptom management.

When it comes to controlling SIBO, self-care is really important. Take part in relaxing and stress-relieving activities, such as yoga, meditation, and time spent in nature. Make time for good coping strategies, frequent exercise, and enough sleep as a way to assist your body's natural healing process. Recall that controlling SIBO is a journey, and your ability to succeed might much depend on your network of support and availability of resources.

Thriving Despite Sibo

Despite the difficulties that come with having SIBO, with the correct care and attitude, it is possible to flourish and have a happy life. Remaining resilient and optimistic amid hardship is essential to living despite SIBO. Concentrate on the things you can manage, such as following your treatment schedule, changing your way of life, and getting help when you need it.

Learning about SIBO and how to treat it is another essential step to living well with this illness. Keep yourself updated with the most recent findings, available treatments, and self-care techniques to take charge of your health. Participate actively in your healthcare journey by speaking up for yourself, asking queries, and, if needed, obtaining second views.

To enhance your general well-being, give priority to holistic methods in addition to medical care. This might include making dietary adjustments, using stress-reduction tactics, and placing an emphasis on self-care routines that uplift your body, mind, and soul. Recall that failures are a typical aspect of the healing process and that progress is not always linear. Acknowledge your progress with grace and acknowledge every modest step you take toward your goals.

In the end, finding perseverance, optimism, and balance amid difficulties is what it takes to thrive despite SIBO. You may maximize your chances of achieving optimum health and well-being by making self-care a priority, building a network of support, and using resources.

CONCLUSION

In summary, a multimodal approach to diagnosis and treatment is necessary for Small Intestinal Bacterial Overgrowth (SIBO), which has a complicated interaction of symptoms and underlying causes. The complex microbial ecology of the small intestine is essential for preserving gut health and general wellness. A disturbance in this equilibrium, either from anatomical irregularities, motility issues, or other risk factors, may cause bacteria in the small intestine to proliferate and eventually cause SIBO.

SIBO may show clinically with a broad range of gastrointestinal symptoms, including diarrhea, bloating, abdominal discomfort, and loss of nutrients. However, because of its generic character, diagnosis is sometimes made more difficult, requiring a mix of imaging modalities, laboratory testing, and clinical suspicion for a correct evaluation.

The goals of SIBO treatment options are to address underlying predisposing factors, eliminate bacterial overgrowth, and restore intestinal motility. The mainstay of SIBO care continues to be antibiotic medication since many medicines have shown promise in lowering the bacterial burden and improving symptoms. To avoid relapse and encourage long-term remission, probiotics, dietary changes, and prokinetic drugs are crucial supplementary therapies. This is because there is a chance of recurrence.

Furthermore, for thorough care and recurrence prevention, it is essential to address predisposing factors such as immunological dysfunction, gastrointestinal motility issues, and anatomical abnormalities. To optimize patient results and provide customized treatment programs, gastroenterologists, dietitians, and other healthcare professionals must work together closely.

In conclusion, a thorough knowledge of the pathophysiology of small intestinal bacterial overgrowth and a multidisciplinary approach to care may greatly enhance patient outcomes and quality of life, even if it presents diagnostic and therapeutic hurdles. To address the changing environment of SIBO management, further research into cutting-edge treatment methods and recurrence prevention tactics is necessary.

THE END

www.ingramcontent.com/pod-product-compliance
Lightning Source LLC
Chambersburg PA
CBHW051908250726

48659CB00002B/544